We Thought We Knew...

Involving patients in nursing practice

Jeanette Copperman
Paula Morrison

Editorial assistance by
Pat Healy

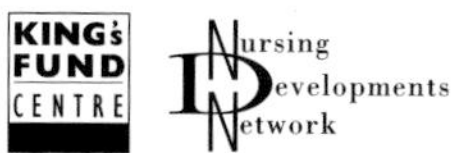

Published by the King's Fund Centre
126 Albert Street
London
NW1 7NF
Tel: 0171-267 6111

ISBN 1 85717 089 X

A CIP catalogue record for this book is available from the British Library

Distributed by:
Bournemouth English Book Centre (BEBC)
PO Box 1496
Parkstone
Poole
Dorset BH12 3YD

The King's Fund Centre is a health services development agency which promotes improvements in health and social care. We do this by working with people in health services, in social services, in voluntary agencies, and with the users of their services. We encourage people to try out new ideas, provide financial or practical support to new developments, and enable experiences to be shared through workshops, conferences and publications. Our aim is to ensure that good developments in health and social care are widely taken up.

Cover photograph: Superstock, Robert Harding Picture Library

Contents

Foreword

The need to hear and take note of the voice of users has received considerable attention in health care over recent years. Yet, in day-to-day practice, ensuring that this is not mere rhetoric but has a real impact on service delivery presents major challenges. Exploring what patients and clients really think about the service they receive requires a creative approach extending well beyond classical patient satisfaction surveys. If we wish to develop a more needs-led, flexible and responsive service then it is crucial that the user's views are sought.

Nurses have always been directly involved in providing care. They are ideally placed to explore the 'real' views of patients about the services they receive, as long as patients perceive nurses as being open and receptive to their concerns. The commitment of nurses to involving patients will be essential in achieving a more user-focused and high-quality service.

The case studies presented in this booklet demonstrate that bringing the voice of users into treatment and service issues changes the perceptions of care givers, and increases patients' confidence in working with professionals. In sharing these experiences, which have arisen from Nursing Development Units in a variety of different settings, many useful lessons have been learned, which may be of help to others. This publication also offers guidelines to practitioners in taking user involvement forward and provides a valuable starting point for debate and action at a local level.

I congratulate all those who have been involved with this work. Their vision and effort have made user involvement a reality in nursing practice. Their experiences need to be shared. It can seem daunting to try to find out and respond to patients' views when there are so many other pressures. This booklet shows how rewarding it can be.

Barbara Stocking
Chief Executive
Anglia and Oxford Regional Health Authority

Acknowledgements

The King's Fund would like to thank the following Nursing Development Units:

Homeward Rehabilitation NDU, Brighton, East Sussex

Stepney Community NDU, Steels Lane Health Centre, London

Tameside and Glossop Mental Health NDU, Ashton under Lyne

Weston Park Oncology NDU, Weston Park NHS Trust, Sheffield

Witney Learning Disability NDU, Witney, Oxon

The willingness of the nurses, managers and advocates to share information, and the time given for interviews and discussion have made this publication possible.

Introduction

The *Patient's Charter*,[1] *Local Voices* [2] and *Caring for People* [3] urge purchasers and providers to take account of health service users and the communities they serve. Since their publication, there have been many policy statements and initiatives at a local and national level which aim to respond to this requirement. Nurses, in day-to-day contact with users, have a key role in turning the rhetoric into reality, but support and information are required to do this.

While the health care reforms heralded a renewed interest in involving users in care, this approach is not totally new. User involvement initiatives have been incorporated in nursing practice in a number of ways for some time. At the provider level, nurses have been involved with giving information to patients, discussing their care with them, responding to their needs and involving them in their own care. The development of primary nursing, care planning and self-medication are examples of a move away from a task-oriented, hierarchical approach to patient/client-focused care. Until recently the term user involvement had not necessarily been used. Patient participation, empowerment of service users, client consultation, even patient-focused care, are a few of the terms that are common to particular settings. While each term implies a certain starting point and approach, in practice they share some underlying principles such as an ethical commitment to respecting people and an attempt to acknowledge people's capacity for autonomy.

Health visitors have focused on involving communities and groups, drawing on techniques from community work, using development approaches which aim to help empower individuals and communities. Notably, midwives in some units have worked with self-help groups and voluntary organisations over a period of years. Thus many changes have taken place in the ways in which maternity services are delivered.[4,5,6,7] There is work to build on, and a need exists to legitimise this work and bring it into the mainstream of nursing practice in a way that is strategic, systematic and makes a difference to the quality of care offered to those who need it. This may enable developments within nursing practice to inform and be linked to initiatives for involving users which are taking place across health care. Such a move is crucial since the involvement of users has been shown to lead to better targeted and more effective outcomes of care.[8]

Models on which user involvement can be based are still evolving. To be effective, information must be collected in a way which allows for changes to be made to the quality of service delivery. To achieve this, McIver[9] suggests that the instruments used must reflect accurately both the views, experiences and opinions of service users and information which relates to issues considered important by service providers. For example, gaining honest feedback from patients can be problematic. Results from patient satisfaction surveys, one of the most common feedback mechanisms in the NHS, show that expressed satisfaction in in-patient wards tends to be as high as 85-90 per cent, but it has been suggested that this relates to feelings of gratitude or vulnerability and is shaped by what is available.[10,11,12] Surveys which concentrate on what actually happened to patients while they were in hospital have been used to provide more accurate information.[13] The resources needed for development and analysis of surveys can, however, be considerable. Open-ended and smaller-scale in-depth studies seem more likely to uncover areas of criticism in the first instance.[14] This is evident from the case studies.

Across specialities, research shows that priorities for users are communication with professionals, quality of treatment and information.[15] To date, much of the user feedback which has been sought in the NHS has related to the hotel and service aspects of care, for example the quality of the physical environment and waiting times. While these are important, raising the status of lay views about the kind of information which is desirable and the preferred methods of communication and treatment needs further development. Traditionally, these have been much more difficult areas to access.

Although there have been increasing enthusiasm and commitment from professionals and there are many initiatives which are gaining momentum, development needs to focus on moving away from the old patient/professional relationships where the practitioners knew best and the patient was the passive recipient of health care. As the case studies in this booklet demonstrate, a new, more questioning environment has emerged which has challenged the old certainties.

Since health care is increasingly perceived to be an inexact science, with large areas of uncertainty,[16] negotiating the status of lay and professional knowledge is being seen as an important way to improve the outcomes of care.[17] This is particularly true among the growing numbers of people with chronic conditions since they see themselves as producers as well as consumers of health care.[18] Much of the work on user involvement and patient participation remains developmental and unevaluated.[19] For example, Glenister[20] in his review of literature on patient participation in mental health services, found that analysis and evaluation of the studies were somewhat lacking in most of the work reviewed. This may be one of the challenges for future work.

To inform the debate, this booklet presents case studies from five nursing development units where the involvement of users and carers is taking place. Some of the units have begun the process relatively recently, such as the Oncology Unit at Weston Park Hospital and Tameside Mental Health Unit, where advocacy was introduced three years ago. Some, like the Witney Unit, have been changing practices and embedding user participation in the organisation over the last ten years. The case studies outlined here are only a few of the initiatives taking place and are only meant to be indicative of much other work which is under way. They were chosen for the range of settings and methodologies which they have employed. They span from Homeward – a rehabilitation ward for older people – to Stepney – a community unit in London's East End. The accounts of managers, advocates and staff illustrate some of the diverse ways in which users have been involved, highlighting the successes achieved and some of the obstacles encountered in developing user involvement initiatives.

As the case studies show, successful user involvement requires a renegotiation of both the individual nurse's role and nursing as a profession within the hierarchy. Enabling front-line staff to challenge existing practices, to question without fear of retribution and to negotiate within the organisational hierarchy were important aspects of creating a climate for change, without which it would have been difficult to take user feedback on board. At the same time, it involved asking nurses to give up aspects of the power they held as professionals and to be open to other very different perspectives. Some of these issues and principles are explored further in section 4 (p.51 ff.) with pointers offered to ways in which user involvement can be taken forward. They are not intended to be exhaustive but a starting point for debate. The case studies illustrate the feasibility of transferring skills and models developed in one setting into another, as long as the models are treated as guides rather than blue prints and adapted flexibly.

User involvement is a vast and developing field. It is not possible to summarise all the issues in one publication, but a list of references is offered at the back of this booklet, and some specialist resources are listed at the end of some of the case studies.

The task of involving users can seem overwhelming, particularly alongside all the other demands that are being placed on provider units. Furthermore, it is not always an easy option, but demands time, resources and commitment. However, the vital ingredients are in place: there is the enthusiasm and commitment to make a concerted effort to bring the voice of users into nursing practice, at all levels.

Guidelines for the introduction of user involvement: a summary

1 Genuine involvement and partnership will take time and commitment to achieve.

2 An awareness of possible constraints to user involvement is needed.

3 All staff, patients, carers and relatives should be offered the opportunity to be involved in the planning of patient participation, recognising that the climate which helps user involvement to flourish is one of partnership and collaboration.

4 Units need management support to implement and to maintain user involvement initiatives.

5 Involving users should take place in both informal and formal ways within organisations.

6 Support, training and resourcing are usually required for user involvement to take place at all levels of the organisation. According to the degree of involvement, both users and staff will need training.

7 Communicating good, relevant information is a prerequisite to user involvement.

8 It is necessary to identify and discuss the ethical dilemmas which user involvement may present in nursing practice.

9 There is no one methodology which is appropriate to all settings. Often a combination of different approaches is most successful. Once the goals of all concerned have been identified, then it is possible to match these with appropriate methods.

10 Work needs to be ongoing, with the relevant results fed back to users and staff. Regular monitoring and evaluation systems should be integral to the process with input from all concerned, including users.

Case Study I

Tameside and Glossop Mental Health NDU
The Tameside Advocacy Service CHAMP (Community and Hospital Advocacy for Mental Health Persons)

About the unit

CHAMP began in September 1991 within the Community and Priority Services, a mental health unit at Tameside General Hospital. The unit includes a day hospital used by up to 60 people a day, an out-patients' department and inpatient wards with 73 beds. CHAMP trains users of mental health services to become advocates for other users, raising complaints and issues about the quality of services.

How it started

The initiative came from service users themselves after a conference on user involvement organised jointly by the local health authority, social services and MIND. They approached staff about the possibility of developing a self-advocacy service. Everyone wanted to give them a voice in how the service that they used was run, and health and social services managers agreed to support the initiative. The service users had also independently contacted other local and national advocacy services and were in the process of establishing a network of support and supervision from independent agencies.

Developing the service

Planning

A steering group was set up to manage the project. It was agreed that service users should fill the key posts of chair and secretary, despite initial doubts. Some managers thought the group should be service-led, while some users felt intimidated at the prospect of chairing a group including managers, doctors, nurses, social workers and representatives of voluntary organisations. It was recognised that the chair and secretary would need organisational and moral support in the initial phase, and this was supplied by a consultant psychiatrist and a senior nurse who were in support of these issues.

Putting it into action

Before CHAMP started work, visits were arranged to other advocacy services to generate interest by users and staff. This was marginally more successful in maintaining interest among users than with staff. CHAMP started work in the day hospital, both because the advocates were using it and because it was the central focus of the different parts of the mental health service. The service later developed to include the outpatient and inpatient wards.

A package of training was developed including counselling, welfare rights and organisational awareness for the advocates.

The project began with an advocate available seven days a week at the day hospital for users experiencing difficulties, who would speak out for them on how the service was run. Two advocates were also invited to join the day hospital's management group that determined policy and strategy.

What it felt like

There were some early difficulties about the status of the advocates. They registered as 'volunteers' to ensure that they were covered by insurance, their expenses could be met, and they would be provided with security badges. But their distinct name badges identified them to users as advocates, not volunteers. Staff were confused by this and taken aback when these 'volunteers' refused to do voluntary work like making teas or doing errands. Staff were also unclear about the advocates' role in the day hospital, with some confusion about when they should be treated as patients and when they were there as advocates.

Some staff initially felt threatened by the advocacy service, perceiving themselves to be under scrutiny by patients. Others felt that advocates had privileges not shared by other patients, while some staff were concerned that advocates knew more than themselves about policy decisions.

Val Wilshaw, one of the advocates, found that the necessary change in culture took time to achieve. She remembers:

'In the beginning they thought I was a spy ... they said "you're always complaining". I explained that I was not complaining for myself, but on behalf of users.'

The initial difficulties were resolved by meetings between managers, staff and advocates which led to a staff/advocate group being set up to share information and develop a climate of partnership. The group met every week with the remit to develop the advocacy service. Meanwhile, the advocates developed their own constitution to define their role and responsibilities, including devising information leaflets for clients and systems for dealing with complaints.

Next steps

Funding came initially from the day hospital budget, but the mental health executive agreed to provide independent finance. This enabled resources to be made available for advocates to run an evening social club from hospital premises, and to establish their own office with equipment, including a dedicated telephone line. They also opened their own bank account to pay for the telephone rental.

Examples of how difficult it was for staff to make the necessary cultural changes include the manner in which the advocates' membership of the mental health executive and the siting of the advocacy office was determined.

An office was identified as suitable for advocacy, sited in the outpatients' department of the unit. There was some resistance to this as it was claimed that medical confidentiality would be compromised. Following negotiation, the office was resited within the administration unit as this maintained the independence of advocacy. Clients also felt it was more appropriate to be seen away from the unit, to maintain their own confidentiality when making complaints. Supervision was offered by the quality adviser who was independent of the mental health unit which promoted advocacy within the framework of service quality.

Staff argued that it would be very confusing for an advocate to attend mental health executive meetings. *'She could not possibly understand all the things we discussed...'* and *'She would need training before she could sit on this group'* were typical comments. Staff were still inclined to be protective towards advocates as they had yet to view them as colleagues rather than patients or ex-patients. Eventually Val Wilshaw was allowed to attend meetings with observer status for a limited period. After a year, when her status was raised, no one opposed her membership.

Outcomes

Advocates rapidly became involved in a variety of projects, including the design and development of a garden for patients which had originally been designated to be a car park, an attendance allowance campaign, petitioning for drinks machines, as well as monitoring the quality of patients' meals. They developed patient information leaflets, surveys and audits of the service.

Their experience of having been psychiatric patients themselves encouraged other users to raise issues and made them less fearful of being critical. They monitored users' views on admission procedures, waiting times, staff attitudes, information, control over treatment and running the services.

Informal afternoon discussion groups facilitated by the advocates were backed up by questionnaires and individual in-depth interviews. Single-sex discussion groups proved more successful because a difference in needs between male and female users was recognised.

This work showed that:

- childcare facilities were a high priority for women users.
- women users wanted to be able to choose single-sex wards.
- when users first arrived on the ward they were often reminded of their first day at school – they were afraid because they did not know simple things like:
  - what was going to happen to them
  - who to ask
  - where the loos were
  - whether they could get a drink
  - what time lunch was.
- users were also afraid of not being believed.
- their problems in sleeping were exacerbated by having to sleep between rubber covers on mattresses and duvets, which made them too hot. This has now been resolved as purchasers have agreed to use duvets without rubber coverings.
- users wanted more information about the side-effects of the medication they were receiving in order to negotiate control over the amount.
- users wanted more privacy and dignity when using washing facilities.

- users felt that their physical complaints were neglected.
- users were critical of relationships with staff.

In response, the unit now gives all new patients an information pack which includes leaflets on advocacy, medication and access to case files. Leaflets encourage users to ask questions.

The advocates represented clients on complaints, housing and benefits appeals and successfully enlisted the support of eight local solicitors who were willing to give free legal advice. They also accompanied clients to see consultants, arranged meetings with key workers and helped them question their care plans, including their medication.

'We could go and explain a panic attack. It is easier for someone who has been there and experienced it to explain it.'

Barriers began to come down when staff saw positive outcomes. The development of a partnership approach achieved changed patterns of work which benefited both staff and users and helped to break down the 'us' and 'them' polarities.

'It has given me my self-esteem back and has done an awful lot for everyone who has been an advocate. Quite a lot have gone on to paid work. Now some of the psychiatrists are suggesting to people that they would make good advocates!'

Advocacy has been successfully developed and is now part of the quality management of the service. Quality managers supervise advocates, who maintain their own independence as members of a separate organisation. Advocates sit on interviewing panels for new staff and comment on candidates' approachability and attitudes to advocacy and complaints.

'The development was not without its difficulties, not least because they were all patients or ex-patients of the mental health services, with all the prejudices and stereotypes this engendered. They had to fight hard and with persistence to maintain both their service and independence.'

The project depended on the commitment of staff and users who spent their free time in the evenings and at weekends attending steering group meetings, and on managers who were prepared to take the risk of developing self-advocacy and providing the resources for it.

'The advocates and staff demonstrated great resilience and commitment to user involvement in what sometimes could be considered a hostile environment. They have battled against prejudice, marginalisation, bureaucracy and themselves. They have developed a partnership with health and social services and have

grown as their service has grown. They have always ensured that the voice of mentally ill people has been heard.'

The main purchasers have now provided joint funding for paid advocacy posts which will be managed by a management committee, including representation from the community health council, the health trust, the social services department, the council for voluntary organisations and representatives of user groups. Advocates are now an integral part of local mental health services.

The project has produced a more questioning culture among both staff and patients. Patients are now more involved and in control of their treatment and the running of the unit. Staff have a better understanding of the effects of mental ill health on patients and their carers, which has helped them to further develop their skills and understanding of those who experience mental health problems.

Lessons learned

'We allowed ourselves to make mistakes and did not blame each other. We accepted when we were defeated on various issues and identified some issues that could be successful to lay the foundation on.' (Alan Slater, Clinical Leader, Tameside NDU)

- To gain support for this kind of project, it is vital to study both how the organisation works and to identify and target key individuals.
- Different levels of support need to be built in at senior and organisational levels.
- It is crucial to acknowledge that there will be difficulties which need to be addressed. To avoid scapegoating and share responsibility for change, this needs to be managed through the group rather than on an individual basis.
- It is important to find ways of getting support from both staff and patients. Those involved in the project found it was necessary to address feelings about preferential treatment through meetings with both.
- It helps to get user representation on to management groups.
- It is useful to acknowledge that raising the status of patients can also empower staff. The low status of psychiatric patients is often reflected on the staff working with them.
- Time is needed to enable advocates to understand how the 'bureaucracy' works.

- While it is impossible to change personalities, behaviour can be altered through changing culture and attitudes.
- Each step has to be negotiated separately, even when everyone supports advocacy in principle.

Issues raised

Advocacy by users offered access to people whose sole qualification was their experience of using services. This challenged the predominant culture of mental health services that users are expected to be compliant.

Senior managers and clinicians broadly supported the advocacy project, but became suspicious when it widened from tackling service issues in the day hospital to medical issues.

Blanket institutional provision was challenged by the advocacy project. Advocates commented that *'a service which is fine for one person is not fine for someone else. Advocacy is about recognising that diversity and getting away from the inflexibility of institutional provision. It is about recognising the rights of the individual.'*

There were constant issues to be negotiated and the success of the project depended on managers and advocates being able to resolve them together, while maintaining the independence of the advocates.

'It is important to have conflict. Very early on we decided to give ourselves the right to make mistakes and the right to disagree with each other and not get on. We also had the unspoken agreement that we could see each other at any time.' (Val Wilshaw, Advocate)

The social club, run by advocates and users, threw up issues about responsibility, for example over making the rules and responding to emergencies. These were resolved through the development of the club's constitution, weekly user/staff meetings and daily informal contacts.

To ensure that advocates could continue to use the hospital services as ordinary users when they needed to, it was formally recognised that they had a 'right to be ill'.

Advocates focused on patients' rights, rather than providing alternative therapy services, although at times patients would disclose sensitive information to advocates that they had not disclosed to their key worker. Constant communication was essential between advocates, patients and staff to enable individuals to discuss issues with their key workers. Supervision was provided for advocates owing to the bombardment, at times, of delicate information disclosed by patients. This demonstrated a need for advocates to be supported by key individuals in the day hospital.

Even though the focus on individual patient rights, and not on challenging the care philosophy, was crucial to the organisational acceptance of the project, conflicts inevitably arose.

The issue of the need for general advocacy services for hospital patients has also been identified through the project. Patients from other parts of the hospital have approached advocates for help and they have taken up cases in children's wards and the older people's unit.

'We learned to leak into the organisation drip by drip, to become part of it, in order to challenge it. Advocacy exploded a lot of myths that professionals have – that they are the only people with the knowledge and the skills, the only people with any creativity and ideas. I was lecturing to students and one of them asked me what my qualifications were. I told him that my qualification was having experienced the services and the good and the bad in them'.

Contributors

Alan Slater, Clinical Leader, Tameside and Glossop Mental Health NDU

Val Wilshaw, Advocate, Tameside and Glossop Mental Health NDU

Useful resource

MIND. The MIND Guide to Advocacy in Mental Health: Empowerment in action. London: MIND, 1992.

Case Study 2

Stepney Community NDU

The new public health approach

'A boy of three told me of his fear of "biters" (cockroaches). He showed me where he had hit the wall with a hammer to kill them. At night he feels safer sleeping under his bed.'

'Two teenage brothers told me of bullying at their school. They said it affected their behaviour and resulted in stomach pains, anxiety and poor school work.'

'Children from a Bangladeshi family said they didn't play by the swings any more as other white children taunted them and threw rubbish.'

'For these children and others like them, their fears have a greater impact on their lives than any other physical effects of socio-economic deprivation. One concerned Bangladeshi father said it was the children's mental health that he worried about most.' (Julia James, clinical leader).

About the unit

Stepney NDU is a community unit with 40 staff, including district nurses, health visitors, school nurses and bi-lingual support workers. The team serve one of the poorest neighbourhoods in the London Borough of Tower Hamlets, which is a multi-cultural area.

The NDU is based on three sites and serves a population of 27,000. More than 30 per cent are Bangladeshi people, 70 per cent of whom are families with children under five. There are at least 20 other races and cultures in the catchment area.

How it started

The frustration of working with individuals who are part of a population experiencing collective hardship and difficulties in getting their health needs met, led nurses to look for different approaches. They were clear that users must be listened to.

Stepney health visitors have described the area as showing many features of inner-city deprivation, including overcrowding in at least a quarter of households and a similar proportion lacking one or more basic amenities. In addition: *'Poor security and isolation are exacerbated by a dearth of community facilities and an inadequate public transport system. Air pollution and dog fouling are rife. Street violence is commonplace. A high unemployment rate, plus poor working conditions and low wages contribute to residents' problems.'* (Savigar & Buxton, 1993)

The Bangladeshi community has particular problems. Their earnings are very low, but racial harassment and tension in the Docklands area have stopped them being rehoused in affordable new housing. The NDU staff believe that poor housing, racism and poverty create *'a social environment which seriously undermines the health of its people.'* (Savigar & Buxton, 1993)

Nurses have also had difficulties in understanding the health needs of those in the local population whose first language is not English. An organisational decision was made to employ Bangladeshi and Somali linkworkers and a Bangladeshi interpreter to help address this issue.

In addition to this, one particular health visiting team employed a bi-lingual Bangladeshi health visitor assistant and, within six months of this appointment, contact between the unit and the Bangladeshi community increased by 400 per cent, and there was a similar increase in the use of local child development screening facilities.

In addition, a health visitor assistant was the first person to discover what was really troubling a newly arrived Bangladeshi woman who was very distressed. Being able to discuss her health with another Bangladeshi woman enabled her to reveal that she was severely depressed and anorexic because she had been incontinent since the birth of her first child 15 months previously.

Developing the service

Planning phase

Stepney NDU decided to adopt a new public health approach to their work. This approach acknowledges both the social and economic factors which undermine and threaten the health of individuals and communities, and the role of health workers as catalysts for change. It stresses the social and political factors affecting health and challenges the traditional boundaries of the service which are based on a medically dominated model. This new approach offers an alternative to the traditional nursing and health promotion practice which emphasises individual lifestyle changes.

It was decided to concentrate on both outreach work and community development to achieve the unit's aims. Instead of expecting people to come into health settings, nurses would visit them in their own communities. They would encourage people to act to bring about change by identifying community priorities and helping to find ways of acting on them.

Putting it into action

The key to this approach was recognised as giving both health professionals and local people an increasing awareness of public health issues. Housing was clearly a major concern, although many other factors affecting public health became a focus of attention.

Stepney health visitors were already aware that housing is a more pressing issue for new mothers than antenatal health. *'They recognise the impertinence of encouraging a mother to make healthy lifestyle changes when her overwhelming concern is how to fit a cot into a bedroom already occupied by six family members or how to keep the cockroaches away from the baby.'* (Savigar & Buxton, 1993)

The NDU staff identified widespread housing problems. Clients faced the barriers of a lack of access to information and professional housing advice when seeking help with their problems. NDU staff felt that this perpetuated their health and welfare problems and interfered with the effectiveness of the care they were providing to their clients. Following consultation with the local law centre, training on the most common housing problems was arranged. This was well attended and spurred the development of a housing clinic attached to a GP group practice. The team successfully identifies and advocates on behalf of those patients suffering the worst housing problems. It has also enabled NDU team members to liaise with local authority departments more effectively through their increased knowledge of the health and housing issues. Future work will concentrate on improving the integration of established health and housing systems.

Next steps

It was realised that ways had to be found of listening to the views of local people, of involving other organisations and of identifying public health issues. For example, the John Smith Children's Centre and

Nursery, the first in the area to be funded by local social services, is now open. The Stepney team intend to be involved in community development initiatives linked with the centre. They are also working with the local East End Mission and the National Children's Home Action for Children charity to develop day care facilities for children with special needs, support for parents, including a crèche, and a community meeting place.

Outcomes

The new approach has resulted in a programme of more than ten projects being set up by the Stepney NDU. They include practical initiatives, such as a health bus which tours estates, markets and community settings with accessible health information, and others aimed at bringing about long-term change to the community. Some examples follow.

ASHA Women's Group

This local Bangladeshi group has provided a focus for health projects in the community. The Bangladeshi linkworker and a health visitor run a joint child health clinic, set up at the group's premises because health care premises were too far away for the mothers to attend. The clinic is an informal, drop-in centre with a crèche, making it much more accessible to local mothers and children.

The women set the agenda for health promotion sessions at the group's premises and invite health workers to come. They have identified food and nutrition as an important health issue. Many Bangladeshi children have feeding difficulties, perhaps because of the tendency to use prepared baby foods, and health visitors are concerned that some toddlers are taking little solid food and are underweight.

A project has been established to look at weaning and feeding infants, and why traditional health promotion methods have not worked with this group. Bangladeshi women and health professionals are reviewing and evaluating the literature, and examining how appropriate the beliefs of health workers are to this group's needs.

At the heart of the project is the acknowledgement that there are different beliefs about food in all cultures. Literature which discusses feeding a baby in a high chair with a spoon is inappropriate for mothers who traditionally use their hands and is going to be rewritten.

The group is also using art to raise the women's self-esteem. Their traditional crafts and skills are being encouraged through the Mogul Tent project, a national embroidery and textile project sponsored by the Victoria and Albert Museum in London. ASHA women will produce one of the panels on the theme of food and nutrition, thus linking directly with the research being undertaken.

Health clinic – quality circle and audit

Building on the work of a quality circle and initial audit, an audit tool is being considered for the child health service. It asks users and professionals for their views on facilities, including access, safety, information sharing, waiting times, transport to and from the centre, opening times and staff attitudes. Long waiting times and lack of space for counselling were identified in one practice as particular problems. As a result, parents and carers are asked to choose whether they want to see the practice nurse, health visitor or GP, which cuts waiting time. A safe play area with play equipment was also set up.

Involving users project

This is an umbrella group for ten active projects with a facilitator and project leader. This project's main task is to find effective ways to consult and involve users of the community nursing service and to ensure that user involvement is built into all NDU projects.

Involvement in small-scale projects has been successful. However, there are still barriers preventing local people becoming more active in the more formal steering group which advises on the overall programme. Local people have found it easier to join smaller local project groups, and this has proved to be much more successful.

Several initiatives aim at raising awareness about the lives of Stepney residents among health professionals. For example, students from a nearby college have made a video entitled *Living in Stepney* in which four local women aged between 16 and 82 talk about their health needs, including housing. Two of the women are Bangladeshi, the others are white East Enders. The video is being shown to students and health workers to stimulate discussion about this population's needs.

Making the video demonstrated some of the difficulties the NDU is experiencing with outreach work. It took six months to make, partly because repeated visits were needed before Bangladeshi families would agree to feature in it. Although health professionals had built up trust with local families, they found it difficult to help Bangladeshi people to recognise that they had valid experiences to share and find the confidence to articulate their views. This is understandable, since they had never been asked before what their views of health care were.

Locally, the video has proved popular, although perceptions about it have differed. Some nurses and health workers have commented that it makes Stepney look more attractive than it actually is, while those working in neighbouring areas said that the poverty stood out.

A follow-up video is in production. It will give 100 local people up to two minutes each to talk about their experiences of living in Stepney, and to say what one thing would make a difference to their health.

Tackling racism

National attention was drawn to Tower Hamlets when a British National Party (BNP) candidate won a council seat in a by-election early in 1994. Although he lost the seat at the subsequent full council elections in May 1994, the impact of a BNP councillor was to produce a highly charged and politicised atmosphere. It was felt important that nurses working in Tower Hamlets had an awareness of these issues.

Student responses to the NDU video of Stepney people demonstrated their lack of insight and knowledge, which mirrors some local attitudes. One student asked on the evaluation form: *'Why do most ethnic communities feel so frustrated about housing conditions? How can we educate them to adopt a western culture if they want a better lifestyle? Why do we have to put up with their problems?'*

Market traders were antagonistic when the health bus visited during National Housing Week. The traders felt excluded by the efforts made by the unit to reach the Bangladeshi community. The need to address historical disadvantage is not often respected.

'The unit is constantly trying to balance different needs and develop practical ways in which health workers can discuss a range of conflicting ideas, safely challenge situations and support families who are experiencing harassment and abuse,' as Julia James, clinical leader of the NDU, says.

Most Bangladeshi families experience racial harassment, although they may use euphemisms to describe it. A woman may tell her health visitor that she does not go out of the house because she has small children, when she may later reveal fears about being attacked. Health workers sometimes feel threatened themselves, as well as powerless to bring about change.

Stepney NDU has been in close contact with a two-year joint FHSA and voluntary sector project looking at the health of recently resettled Bangladeshi and Somali homeless families. This project has identified racial harassment as a major health issue for these families. It has now developed into the Resettlement Advocacy Project (RAP) which has carried out a series of workshops with community nursing staff in the Isle of Dogs, looking at how primary health care staff experience racism through their work. This project intends to encourage similar developments in other primary health care teams and to produce standardised procedures for use by primary health care workers district-wide who are dealing with racial harassment at managerial, professional and user levels. The Stepney NDU is keen to develop this training by taking up the model being developed by RAP of providing continuing support for staff on the issue of racism.

Tackling such issues is integral to the philosophy of the Stepney NDU and inevitably requires multi-agency links.

Children's rights

The NDU is working on a children's public and mental health project. This aims at helping children to become empowered by consulting them, sharing information with them and encouraging them to state their own points of view. A large proportion of the NDU service users are children. Julia James, clinical leader of the NDU, questioned them at home and at school about what distressed them, and they talked about *'big dogs, nowhere to play, racism, scary people.'*

The project includes the development of standards on children's consent to treatment and ensuring that they are always greeted by name. A video is planned in which children will talk about the area they live in and how it affects their lives.

Older people

Teams of workers are being encouraged to identify public health issues, and this has led to traffic and transport problems being identified as concerns for older people who rarely go out. They were afraid to cross roads with fast-moving traffic, experienced difficulties in accessing Dial-a-Ride, and needed guidance on how to deal with bogus callers so that they could answer the door safely.

Young people

The NDU is working with other agencies to tackle issues of sexual health, safety and drugs from the perspective of Bangladeshi youths on a run-down estate. This work is linked to national and local *Health of the Nation* targets.

District nurse documentation

Patients hold the records used by district nurses, but seldom use them themselves. A simple record that could be used by clients, carers and other health workers is being developed in partnership with clients. It will include a 'social map' and local information. Most users are still not confident about writing in their records, however. A drug chart that can be read and understood by clients will be incorporated into the notes. This initiative links with local continuing care and discharge policies and is being developed in conjunction with acute services.

The future

The success of an initial focus group for women who had or have leg ulcers led to plans for regular meetings for users. This provided a forum for mutual support and sharing of experiences. The focus group of the well-leg project generated a community campaign involving a poster which aimed at getting people to seek professional help earlier.

The nurses at Stepney NDU have realised how valuable this user perspective has been. It has led to the well-leg project being revised in order to reflect users' views, which in turn has contributed to improved outcomes of care. Stepney NDU plans to use the approach of focus groups to gain user perspectives in other projects within the service.

Lessons learned

Consultation with users in Stepney has demonstrated that users are not homogeneous and their interests do not always coincide. These differences must be reflected in methods of consultation. Large open forums may not be appropriate.

Racism and issues about the representation of black communities exist in all other communities and are openly acknowledged in Stepney. Working in different gender and race groups is an effective way of giving black communities a voice.

Issues raised

The importance of multi-agency work in tackling health issues in areas like Stepney has been demonstrated by the NDU's work with lawyers on housing problems, with voluntary agencies on child care and with practice nurses and GPs on child development work.

Employing people from minority ethnic communities who can communicate with local people in a common language enables a range of previously unknown health needs to be identified, particularly around women's health.

Discriminatory professional attitudes need to be challenged so that all cultures and lifestyles are respected on their own terms.

User involvement needs to become a way of life for health workers and not just a targeted activity.

The question raised most often in response to Stepney NDU's work has been: *'Is this nurses' work?'* The team believes it is not possible to consider health issues in Stepney out of the context of the extreme deprivation of the area.

'It has to be nurses' work in an area like this. If we do not address poverty and deprivation, then we cannot address health need.'

Contributor – Julia James, Clinical Leader, Stepney NDU.

Useful resources

James J. Application for Children's Rights in Nursing Award. RCN/Gulbenkian award, 1994. (Unpublished)

James J. Literature Review on Child Empowerment Models and Their Application to Health Visiting. (Unpublished)

Savigar S, Buxton V. Grasping the nettle. Primary Health Care 1993; 3:5.

About the unit

Witney NDU works with people with severe learning disabilities of all ages. The work on improving choice in their everyday lives was pioneered in three residential houses on the same site. The residents are predominantly male and most have little verbal communication, although the majority have developed their own communication systems. A few also have physical disabilities. For a lot of these clients continuing help with everyday tasks is needed.

Although the houses were closer to community facilities than the old institution, the number of people living in each house was too high, eight in fact, with people sharing bedrooms. In reality, all that had happened was that the large institution had been replaced by three mini-institutions. Over the past year, residents have moved again to four purpose-built houses in order to create the opportunity for a more normal lifestyle. The work on improving choice continues in these houses.

How it started

Jamie Shephard, clinical leader, says *'work began on choice several years ago. In fact, the work on choice stems from a bottle of tomato sauce or, should I say, the lack of one. I was having a meal with people who live in residential accommodation for people with a learning disability. It was fish and chips for lunch. I always have ketchup with my chips – there was no sauce on the table, although there were several bottles in the cupboard in the kitchen. How did staff know if someone wanted ketchup? It was maybe not a question of choice being denied but opportunities for choice not being realised.'*

The move from an institution in the middle of the countryside to purpose-built houses next to local community facilities, including the post office and shops, had not brought many changes in nursing practice. Managers, senior nurses and direct care staff were given a mere two-week preparation prior to the move from the institution to community facilities.

This meant that institutional practices continued. The residents would be up and dressed at 6.30 am and face a day in which meals were not social events. Breakfast was over in a few minutes, the midday meal was from 11.30 to noon, and the evening meal at 4 pm.

Basic hygiene and medical needs were met and people were well fed, but it was block treatment with little flexibility or individual choice. Residents would go to bed at 8 pm when the night staff arrived. Clothes would be washed at night and put in bundles by their beds for use the next day, giving residents little choice about what to wear.

'We were starting from the very basics of choice.'

Developing the service

Improving choice

Three new senior nurses were recruited to work on improving the services offered to the clients. Emphasis was placed on team building, with help from outside educators facilitating team-building days.

There was a need to address very basic issues, and standard setting was identified as a valid method to bring about change.

'We started with the use of toilets. In each of the houses there were three toilets, and there was an unwritten rule that one of them was the staff toilet. The first standard we set was that residents could use any toilet. The idea was to bring the rest of the toilets up to the standard of the staff toilet. Obviously, that had huge implications for people who had worked in institutions and were used to segregation. There was rejection of the ideas and a lot of confrontation.'

Other standards were set for meal times, for when people got up and went to bed, for how residents would interact with the local community. Residents were also given the opportunity to help make their own meals and to choose their own clothes. Early work provided opportunities for people who could not communicate verbally to make their own choices. At the same time, staff were encouraged to think about why things were done in a particular way.

Putting it into action

The nurses employed to change practice felt that there was a need for those staff working with residents to realise and understand that people with little or no verbal communication skills could make their needs and feelings known through non-verbal expression, including signs, hand signals and varying voice tones.

Activity charts were used to identify opportunities for choice and to encourage staff to review block treatment critically. Awareness-raising was used to teach staff about the importance of giving people with learning difficulties opportunities to make mistakes, to experience a range of emotions and to take risks.

'It was about a change in culture. We all realised that the previous practices were no one's fault. In the past, the only input from a senior nurse had been inspecting beds to make sure they were properly made. If a staff member was seen talking to a resident and there was an unmade bed, they would have been told off. We tried to reverse that and say, 'It's OK to just sit and talk to people'. In fact, it is really important. To stop them tidying up all the time was difficult. If they did practical tasks, they could see what they achieved. Talking to somebody is much harder to measure.'

What it felt like

Care staff, nurses and residents reacted in different ways. A crucial issue was persuading care staff to allow nurses to introduce changes. Care staff were mainly female, had no professional training and had been largely left to get on with it. For most of them it was the first time that they had negotiated with senior nurses about their work. If the changes were to be successful, getting care staff to discuss what standards should be set and how they would affect practice was more important than the standard setting itself.

Care staff eventually felt able to raise issues related to practice, in respect to clients and communication with senior nurses. Sensitive issues such as sexuality were tackled. This and other issues demanded both honesty and the ability to tolerate discomfort.

Nurses helped to develop care staff to this stage in a number of different ways. A key strategy was using role models. The development team worked in each of the three houses, demonstrating how nurses believed the services should be provided. The initial response from care staff was unfavourable; they said the nurses were *'half bonkers'* and thought they would not last.

Team work enabled people to identify the need to be honest and open, which led staff to prioritise issues which were worked on jointly. Nurses felt that more could be achieved by setting local standards for each of the three houses. That enabled a sense of ownership with the clients and care staff so that more complex standards could be developed around issues such as who should be responsible for answering the door and the telephone.

People without verbal communication should not be excluded from those responsibilities and ways had to be found of including them. Residents realised this did give them more choices, including declining to answer the door or telephone if they were busy doing something else.

One of the successful strategies for gaining ownership of the changes was the positive changes staff saw in clients who had moved from the old institution.

'People had initially to be sedated to make the move from Bradwell Grove because they had not been out before. Now they were going out in the car and going out to the shops. Staff saw those positive changes in someone they had known for thirty years.'

Next steps

Plans were made to move the residents into more suitable accommodation in the community. The three existing houses were sold and the proceeds used to buy four houses, of which two were purpose-built with adaptations for people with physical disabilities. Aware of the mistakes made in relation to the move from the large institution to the initial community setting, it was vital that as well as the clients moving into 'nicer and more appropriate accommodation', nursing practices were developed, which led to greater choice being offered resulting in greater empowerment for the client. Therefore new homes were located within a community, enabling a more 'normal' lifestyle to be achieved. The needs and wishes of residents were assessed before they moved to their new homes and efforts were made to match residents with each other and with care staff with similar interests.

Outcomes

Developing choice

Some residents were limited by their physical disabilities in making everyday choices. A 'switch' system was therefore introduced enabling residents to turn on equipment, such as lights, television and radio. Initially designed to help one resident to become more active, the switch system is being developed further; however, raising funds for the manufacture of equipment appropriate to people with both physical and learning disabilities has proved difficult.

The work in fostering individual choice has developed into group work, with nurses encouraging residents to jointly express their needs and link up with other groups. A graphic complaints procedure with step-by-step pictures has emerged from this.

An empowerment group has been set up, with support from the Trust. This has brought clients from across the county to meetings which aim at setting guidelines for staff on how the service can be run sensitively. An early issue raised by the group was the tendency for staff to walk away during a conversation. Therefore guidelines have been developed by clients on the issue of listening.

The empowerment group has linked up with well-established self-advocacy groups, which may be accessing services from private organisations or from social services. This link is vital because social services are responsible for inspecting health authority homes. The NDU hopes service users will become involved in these inspections and steps are being taken to this end.

'Rather than professionals asking people what they want, people in self-advocacy groups who are used to living in residential accommodation come and ask the questions. They know what it is like to get a cold cup of tea. They pick up things that social services people won't because they do not have the experience.'

Getting people with learning disabilities to talk to each other and represent each other has demonstrated that, although they are often isolated, they have common problems because of their experiences. Some found it hard to cope with the choices that became open to them after years of having all their decisions made for them. It was also difficult for staff to let go in order to give residents genuine choice. Thus developing ways to improve choice has taken a long time and has required a great deal of input from clients, senior nurses, care staff and managers.

This can arise, for example, over holidays. Most people with learning disabilities were used to going to either Butlins or places that specialise in catering for them as a group. But the new era of choice has opened up the possibility of holidaying abroad. If a trusted member of staff tells a resident that he/she would 'love to go to Spain', the choice for the resident may be immediately limited because the resident may feel he/she should choose Spain because of the trust built up between them. It was realised that a more meaningful choice would be offered by bringing in several holiday brochures or by changing the way questions are posed, being aware of tone of voice and facial expressions. The difficulties of being impartial when offering people real choices highlights the skills needed for this type of interaction to truly take place.

'It is very hard not to pass on your own perceptions of life and your own likes and dislikes to someone you have some control over. For example, someone of my age may want to wear denims, but someone in their 50s might want to wear a suit. In the old days, everybody used to wear what the charge nurse wore. If the charge nurse smoked, then all the clients smoked. You would go on to a ward, and there would be ten people all dressed the same way as the charge nurse, smoking.'

Managing money has been another issue that needed consideration to achieve choice for residents. Previously, hospital residents had to queue up to ask for access to their own allowances and were given credit notes for shopping. Now residents have been introduced to budgeting and will, with safeguards, be able to hold their own bank accounts.

A higher education input, student placements and various training courses were all used to introduce new practices. Work continued on breaking the standards down to house level, with the ultimate aim of setting individual standards for each resident. This helped in attaining ownership by staff and clients for the practice changes.

Gradually practice is moving closer to that. One resident's recent bereavement and close relationship with a staff member highlighted the need for staff to allow residents to grieve and to be able to recognise the emotional impact of bereavement for people without verbal communication. The need to grieve has often been overlooked in people with learning disabilities, but now it has been recognised and worked at.

Sexuality presents complex and sometimes controversial issues. One man who had a profound disability showed the need to express his sexuality. A standard was set about this which had a profound effect on the staff.

'Most of the care staff were middle-aged women and we were saying you need to accept that this man wants a blue video, or an adult magazine or book. How do you address and deal with that? That is where you get into very complex needs that are related to someone's choice.'

One of the lessons learned from the process was the importance of individual support for staff members as well as team building.

'If you are raising issues like sexuality, then all staff, including care staff, need regular structured supervision where they get the opportunity to talk about the effect it is having on them, the way they perceive it, how things are changing. Staff can end up feeling disempowered and you cannot carry through changes without them. The biggest percentage of input to the client on a day-to-day basis is from unqualified staff.'

Getting together

'We had people from a highly skilled self-advocacy group who have been together for quite a few years come over and meet some of the clients in a pub and chat to them about what they wanted from the service. Just people talking to each other.'

The value of people with learning disabilities meeting each other, as well as integrating into the rest of the community, is very important. If people are not encouraged to meet and take on pressure group roles, they become very isolated in small groups, although there are a lot of common themes. Because of the drive towards normalisation and community integration that tends to be forgotten. Partly this is a move towards re-establishing those links and getting people to talk to each other, to be represented by other people with a learning disability.

'The importance of a step-by-step approach to empowerment and an approach which allows for individual difference was stressed. When it came to giving choice, after years of having everything decided for them, people were being expected to make decisions for themselves. Some people found that hard to cope with. You have to start with the basic choices, with people getting used to making those small but very important decisions – do they want tea or coffee? It is really the process of giving people the opportunities to be involved, a lot of beginning work needs to be done prior to those levels of group involvement.'

Communicating in different ways

One of the clients is now actively involved in a service user group run by social services. This person has no verbal communication but is able to communicate in other ways. He is making his own video, so that he can communicate with others about his environment in order to make people aware of what can be offered to people with learning disabilities.

Independence

The need for independence in any kind of audit was stressed by the NDU. The fear of victimisation for those who are in receipt of any kind of service has been well documented, particularly for people in residential accommodation. Acknowledging how hard it is for people to be critical about aspects of their environment when they are dealing with people who make decisions on their lives, the NDU and social services are looking at the possibilities of exchanges with residents from elsewhere in the country. The importance of good links between the health authority and social services and the other disciplines was highlighted as critical.

The work of the NDU has led to increased independence for service users, a better quality of life and improved communication skills. On a basic level, residents can now decide whether they would prefer to listen to music or to watch television. Greater changes in behaviour have occurred too, but these small indicators can be just as significant to the people concerned.

One resident who had been labelled as showing *'challenging behaviour'* is now described as a changed man. He used to hit other residents regularly or smash windows out of frustration, which raised the issue whether it was an acceptable risk to allow him to go to the training centre on his own each day despite his deteriorating eyesight. The route meant crossing several roads. Offering this man choices, autonomy and empowering him have meant that his violence has subsided. Recognition that he needed his own space led to his bedroom being turned into a bedsit, allowing him time and space to collect his thoughts. His views were listened to and he now accesses work on his own.

Lessons learned

The importance of continuity of relationships between staff and residents was evident, and having a stable workforce was important to be able to offer that. For example, the maintenance of relationships between clients and staff who may no longer work within the NDU is seen as vital. Both clients and staff are encouraged to maintain links.

In retrospect, although the NDU did a good deal of team building with staff, more structured individual support throughout the process of change would have been helpful.

'You have to be prepared to support individual staff through the process, they will not know what to expect'.

Keeping a record of what you have achieved, the difficulties and the challenges will help you to share your experiences with others.

'Write it down as you go, so that it can be shared with other people. There is a need to know for yourself where you have come from and where you are going to.'

Issues raised

It is important to have the right skill mix and appropriate training for staff. Done properly, this is not a cheap option.

Conflict will arise and staff must be prepared for it. This makes collaboration essential with nursing colleagues as well as care staff. The key to dealing successfully with conflict and maintaining the energy to continue making changes was offered by providing enough support from both co-workers and managers. Having a supportive management style was essential if things were to change and to help maintain the stamina to keep making changes.

The lead and support came from management who brought in dynamic change agents. In this instance it was change from the top, and therefore collaboration with colleagues was essential in ensuring that the work continued.

'Giving people choice means professionals losing some kind of authority and it does present risks. So there are a lot of people saying we are not doing that because it is a health and safety risk, we need to lock the kitchen door because so and so does not wash his hands before he touches food ... the unions become involved.'

The ultimate argument that people use against offering choice is to say *'well at the end of the day they haven't got much choice at all!'* To some degree their argument is correct. However, the same can be said for any of us. Decisions are made over which we may have little or no control. Professionals make decisions they honestly believe to be correct. This only highlights all the more the importance of giving basic choices to people when the opportunity arises.

Realistic expectations

There is an expectation that when a unit is labelled an NDU they have reached some unbelievably high standard of practice, but in reality most of the work is very basic.

This work is ongoing and still evolving, needing constant re-evaluation.

Contributors

Jamie Shephard, Clinical Leader, Witney Learning Disability NDU
Michael Hill, Acting Clinical Resource Manager

Useful resources

Brechin A, Swain J. Changing Relationships. Shared Action Planning with People with a Mental Handicap. London: Harper and Row, 1986.

Crawley B. What Is Self-Advocacy? London: CMH, 1988.

Garbit R, Shephard J. Developing choice. Nursing Times 1993; 89:12.

Hersovj J. Advocacy Issues for the 1990s. In Thampson T, Mathias P (eds). Standards and Mental Handicap. Keys to competence. London: Bailliere Tindall, 1992.

Williams P, Shoultz B. We Can Speak for Ourselves. Self-advocacy by mentally handicapped people. London: Souvenir Press, 1982.

Case Study 4
Weston Park Oncology NDU
Using focus groups

'The important thing to establish is a culture where patients are encouraged to ask questions.'

About the unit

Weston Park is a supra-regional centre for oncology and radiotherapy in Sheffield. Ward 3 serves 27 patients with a diagnosis of cancer, whose treatment includes intensive nursing, chemotherapy, radiotherapy and surgery. Biological and metabolic studies are also carried out on the ward.

'The treatment needed by patients is often complicated and initially difficult for people to accept, not least because of the many side-effects encountered. This, together with the devastating effect that a diagnosis of cancer has on patients and their families, may create an image of a ward where distress and depression are prevalent. This is far from true, and is regarded as one of the many myths the team on the ward has worked hard to dispel.'

How it started

The unit has a history of valuing innovation by nursing staff and encouraging the development of new ways of working. The team wanted a comprehensive evaluation of their work which would reflect the views of staff and patients.

'Past experiences had demonstrated that considerable improvement can be made from quite small innovations, many of which are greatly valued by patients. However, without detracting from the value of many of the improvements made, we, as a team, had to face the fact that most of them had been implemented because we – the nursing staff – felt that the patients would benefit from them! Our perceptions were the result of much patient interaction but, until last year, there had been no formal means of addressing changes wanted by patients themselves, or how they valued the services offered to them.'

Developing the service

Planning phase

Non-nurse consultants were commissioned to run a series of independent focus groups with patients as part of the NDU's aim of improving the quality of care. Patient satisfaction questionnaires were already routine within Weston Park but it was recognised that these only offered one perspective. The team wanted the ward to be evaluated more fully from the patients' perspective. Through patients using their own words it was hoped that this would highlight both areas of satisfaction and where there was room for change.

Hospital staff were excluded from taking part in these focus groups in order to encourage honest criticism from patients, who might otherwise feel they were being disloyal to ward staff.

Putting it into action

A cross-section of patients were selected on age, sex, disease and treatment criteria, and invited to join group discussions on how they felt about the ward environment and their care. Sessions took place in a separate meeting room and were scheduled to last no more than 30 minutes. Groups were encouraged to be honest about the good and bad aspects of their care in order to help plan changes and improvements.

The groups were led by a facilitator who talked about her impressions of visiting Weston Park for the first time and her preconceived ideas. She asked members of the groups to say how they had felt when first admitted to the 'cancer hospital'. She was asked to cover some specific points in the discussions, including what patients thought about self-medication and what they understood by 'complementary therapy'. The role of the focus groups was also to open up free discussion on any topics concerning the care they received or would like to receive in the future. Topics covered included admission procedures, the quality of nursing care, complementary therapies, self-medication and access to patient records.

Five group discussions were held on the ward over a three-week period, and the views of 20 people were obtained, including two carers. More severely disabled patients were included by being interviewed at their bedsides.

Two separate staff focus groups were held for nurses and support staff to give their views about the quality of care, how they thought it could be improved, and to identify areas where patient and staff perceptions differed or agreed.

What it felt like

When and how information should be given and how to involve patients in decision making about their own care can raise a number of dilemmas for nurses in this setting. It is recognised that receiving a diagnosis of cancer can leave people feeling frightened and vulnerable. Nurses felt that a great deal of skill and judgement was needed when considering informed consent to treatment. Together with this there was the realisation that organisational constraints may deter changing certain situations that were of concern to patients.

However, patients' wishes must be the driving force for development, in order that the service offered is, as far as possible, tailored to their individual needs.

Next steps

The focus groups produced positive feedback from patients on the quality of attention they received.

'It was nice to get good feedback about general things – that the atmosphere was friendly and the staff were approachable. But some things really surprised us.'

Not everything was positive. The focus groups identified a number of issues on which patient care could be improved. A key point was the need to improve the information given to patients at each stage of their treatment.

There is a plan to form new focus groups to look at the needs of adolescents in this setting. An initial questionnaire showed that 50 per cent of those questioned would like to be in a separate unit with their own common room. It is hoped that by continuing these groups the users will have greater involvement in decisions regarding the service they receive and its developments, thus realising user involvement in practice.

Outcomes

As a result of the information gleaned from the focus groups, several changes are under way.

Information

Patients who were already self-medicating showed considerable support for it. One commented: *'It makes you feel less helpless and saves nurses' time.'* But others were less sure. They asked why nurses were not giving the medication: *'Isn't it part of their job?'* This disparity was tackled by increasing the amount of written information about self-medication for patients, with separate information sheets being prepared for nurses and doctors. This particularly helped junior doctors who were new to both oncology and self-medication. The practice has now been extended to other wards.

Informing patients that they have a right to see their own medical records has been seen as a priority since the focus groups identified that some patients thought they were not allowed to do so. This suggests that changes in practice are still needed if some patients feel they need permission from medical staff before they can read their own notes. Patients who knew they could do so expressed satisfaction about their medical records.

Involving patients in decision making about their own care may prove more difficult. Most people in the focus groups said that their treatment had been explained at every stage, but some felt they wanted more information, particularly about drugs and their side-effects. The unit has its own library and maintains links with voluntary organisations and self-help groups. Finding the best way of informing and empowering users about how different interventions will affect them often raises ethical dilemmas for staff. It is therefore essential to have staff support mechanisms.

Nurses feel it is particularly important to obtain informed consent to treatment owing to the fear and vulnerability created by a diagnosis of cancer. In the past, women with breast cancer were sometimes asked the night before their operation to choose between a lumpectomy or a mastectomy. They would turn to the nurse to ask what they should do. In order to prevent such occurrences, counselling is now offered at peripheral clinics along with improved information.

The important thing is to give choice, which means helping patients to understand the implications of their disease. That involves giving them the information they need by encouraging them to ask questions, but requires very skilful nursing.

Practice changes

The focus groups now form part of the overall philosophy of care. Standard setting and audit are ongoing within the ward. Nursing staff prioritise the standards to be worked on in relation to the information gathered through the focus groups and carry out their own audits.

There was unexpected feedback from patients about complementary therapies which were in use before the study began. Patients said that they relieved tension and boredom and commented that it was nice to be pampered. They particularly valued the time nurses spent at the bedside giving complementary therapies during long periods of the day when they were in bed or movement was limited by intravenous therapies. This led the team to consider how the presence of nurses at the bedside could be increased as well as improving training in complementary therapies.

More information on specific therapies like massage is now given, and patients have been given relaxation tapes which they can listen to on headsets. The team now feel that when patients ask for a nurse to help them relax, it may indicate a need for a discussion about the fears and worries they may have. Further work is continuing on the use and effectiveness of such therapies.

The team have not yet found a way of resolving how to reduce the anxiety of patients who are disturbed by seeing other severely ill patients when they first arrive on the ward. Side rooms are already offered to very ill patients for their own privacy, but not all accept them.

The unit is now developing an ethical model for involving patients with cancer in decision making about their involvement in randomised controlled trials (RCTs). The prospect of taking part in such trials can raise false hopes for patients and the nurses are examining this issue further with users.

Involving users in care planning is key to the philosophy of treatment, but requires skill and judgement. Where care plans include chemotherapy and radiotherapy treatments, the plan itself provides a focus for discussing them. But where patients are still in denial, it is particularly difficult for nurses to find ways of involving them in care planning. This is so even when the treatment is palliative rather than curative. Care plans need to have factual statements about diagnosis and treatment. Sometimes, those requirements offer the opportunity to open up discussion, but they can also add pressure to an already vulnerable patient. It is critical that patients retain the right to decide not to know what is happening to them.

Patients identified squeaky shoes worn by night staff and the uncomfortable and sweaty plastic linings under pillow-cases as causes of broken sleep. These were simple issues, but staff had been unaware of them before. The pillow-case issue was resolved by patients suggesting they bring in their own pillows – and some now occasionally bring in their own duvets as well.

Admission changes

Better admission procedures to relieve patients' anxiety and save time were identified as priorities. The admission section, medical records and pharmacy now liaise to ensure that patients are given appropriate admission appointment times. Most patients are receiving chemotherapy, and this simple change has reduced their waiting time for a bed from six hours to one, which has had a major impact on reducing anxiety and frustration.

The focus groups findings also showed that patients were given too little information about what to expect before they were admitted to hospital. The hospital is now planning to send out more information about its general policies, but specific information about the individual patient's treatment cannot be offered until the particular procedure that is to be used is decided. As soon as this information is available the issues can be discussed with patients so that their worries can be aired and addressed.

There was a high degree of agreement between the patient and staff focus groups, particularly on the need to improve admission procedures, to give more information about self-medication, and the quality time, including physical touch, which nurses could give through administering complementary therapies. The importance of involving all staff and valuing their contributions has been integral to the work.

The future

Originally planned as a 'one off' exploratory study, focus groups are now integral to the work of the ward. Information from them will be fed into the standard-setting and audit processes. Interviews with out-patients who have left the ward are also being considered to feed into further development.

Lessons learned

The use of focus groups has allowed patients to have greater involvement in decisions regarding the service that they receive and its developments.

Future developments will become more patient-focused through asking patients what they would like to see change.

Some issues concerning patients were simple to address – for example, changing the pillow covers to allow a more comfortable sleep had a dramatic effect on patient satisfaction. Other issues implied further questions and brought to the surface the ethical dilemmas faced in practice. It must be remembered that patients themselves can sometimes offer alternative answers to some of these questions.

Issues raised

The difficulties of involving night staff, who are separate from day staff, need to be addressed even when a ward has a history of encouraging innovative practice. Standard setting can be used to address such issues. At Weston Park, standards on better nurse documentation involving night and day staff have been developed and have been found to be an effective way of responding to this need.

User involvement can be carried out on an acute ward where both palliative and curative medicine is being used. This may raise particular ethical concerns about when and how to raise difficult issues. Information giving in this setting requires sensitive skills and judgement, allowing patients to choose what they would like to know.

Qualitative work with patients may be difficult to measure in ways that satisfy purchasers, who may be more interested in quantitative measures, such as a reduction in the number of pressure sores. However, focus group results could be given to purchasers to inform them of users' views.

Contributor

Ruth Logan, Clinical Nurse Leader, Weston Park Hospital. Sheffield.

Useful resource

Logan R. Focusing on Users. KF News 1994; 17:1.

Case Study 5

Homeward Rehabilitation NDU

Involving patients in their rehabilitation

'We thought we understood how patients felt, we thought we knew the problems they were experiencing, but everyday the patients came up with things we had not thought about. It is a very humbling experience.'

About the unit

Homeward is a 22-bed rehabilitation unit for older people in Brighton. Four beds are designated for people who have had an amputation; the rest are for people who have suffered a stroke, people with neurological disease, arthritis or problems with post-operative recovery. The average stay on the ward is three months.

How it started

Some years ago several nurses, including two sisters, started work on the ward within a short time of each other. They were appalled by the conditions they found and were determined to make changes. As a mark of things to come, the unit was renamed the Homeward Unit.

Homeward is housed in a former workhouse. It was a long-stay elderly unit in Brighton General Hospital until 1984 when it was redesignated as a rehabilitation unit. Some of the conditions as late as the 1970s were graphically described by Barbara Sheppard in her book *Looking Back – Moving Forward*. The following extracts are based on interviews with nurses who worked on the continuing care unit.

'The physical environment remained extremely poor. The walls had not been painted for many, many years and when it rained nurses in one notorious ward had to put buckets around the ward to catch the leaks. The wards stank like a cesspit not only of urine and faeces but also of gangrene, which was very prevalent.'

'Many of the patients had been in hospital for many years and had become utterly institutionalised, losing all individuality. To the staff they seemed merely "human blobs". Most never spoke at all and at least half of them had to be spoon-fed.'

Despite the ward's redesignation, there was little rehabilitation input, and it was regarded as a 'holding bay' for older people while the consultant decided what to do with them. It was not an environment conducive to preparing older people to be independent.

As a first step nurses set up a quality circle which highlighted the poor environment, but matters were brought to a head by a death on the ward.

'As usual, the porters, unable to bring the mortuary trolley along the corridor, had had to wrap the body in a sheet and carry it the length of the ward'.

This was a distressing situation for both patients and staff, and the nurses decided that immediate and drastic action was needed to change this situation. The nurses decided to show how dangerous the ward environment was by removing all patients from the ward while staff and volunteers simulated a fire. At last there was agreement by managers to fund environmental upgrading. This was the start of the many changes needed in order to facilitate development in rehabilitation services.

'Elderly care was seen as not important, and that worked to our advantage. At the same time as the upgrading went on, there were a lot of initiatives that no one knew about. As nurses, we were allowed to manage ourselves and change practices.'

Developing the service

Involving the patients

'Patients were told that they were coming to a rehabilitation unit, and they envisaged some brilliant new unit which was very modern. What they actually came to was the old workhouse. It was dilapidated with paint peeling off the walls and although it had some dynamic people working in it, they identified the workhouse as the place you came to die.'

The staff recognised that patients must be more involved if rehabilitation was to be made more therapeutic. The first step was to find out what patients wanted. Initially, most of the issues raised were about the poor environment which restricted the independence the unit was trying to encourage.

'They had spent a lot of money building a gym which was in the building but not on the same level as the ward … patients had to go downstairs for

rehabilitation as if it was completely separate from what went on in the ward. We wanted to make the whole environment more therapeutic.'

A more patient-centred philosophy of care was drawn up focusing on patients' needs, rather than nursing tasks.

'It seemed obvious but it had not been done. It meant going back to the patients and saying, "how much involvement do you want? Where do you think you could be involved?".'

Putting it into action

A more informal approach was introduced after a presentation on primary nursing for patients, visitors and friends. Nurses stopped wearing uniforms, a member of staff brought a dog onto the ward, and people were given more choice about their daily programmes – for example, deciding when they got up and dressed. The aim was to produce a more home-like environment.

'In the old model of rehabilitation, patients were told what to do. They were not given the idea they had some part to play in it. Rehabilitation was seen as a passive thing.'

The nurses' role was redefined as supporting patients to become independent spiritually, emotionally and physically. Nurses adopted a philosophy of care that meant asking patients what they thought. Nevertheless, they knew that there was still a long way to go.

'We were still working in very traditional ways. The physiotherapists would do their bit, the occupational therapists their bit, patients were grateful to the doctors for "making us better". The nurses' role was perceived as getting patients ready for the therapists, yet we felt we were also therapists and the patients were with us 24 hours a day.'

What it felt like

The development of primary nursing enabled nurses to form closer relationships with patients.

'We began by talking to patients on an informal basis. Then we tried suggestion boxes, but they just got filled with sweet wrappers! We realised early on that patients feel very threatened and vulnerable on the ward. When you asked, "What do you think?", they always answered, "You are wonderful! You are so busy." That was worrying – that they always thought we were too busy. Consultation was still very superficial.'

Homeward has meant a major transition for nurses used to working in more traditional ways. Acknowledging that users have their own values and desires means extra responsibility, which has been both a welcome and a frightening change particularly for staff used to uniforms and fixed roles. Unlike their previous experience on other wards, nurses were encouraged to be involved with all aspects of a patient's recovery. Some found the changes too difficult and left. Yet, the positive outcomes outweigh this loss. Nurses have found themselves empowered through involving users. Because patients wanted to know when their own primary nurse would be on duty, a new roster system was introduced to allow the nurse to be there during the patient's ward round. The weekly roster was given to patients, which meant that patients could negotiate with nurses about off-duty and flexi-time hours.

Nurses were very positive about the way innovation was welcomed on Homeward and found the culture markedly different from more traditional approaches. As they report: *'Several people still found it amazing that they could speak frankly without fear of either aggression or condemnation.'* (Sheppard, 1994)

The management style of the clinical leader was crucial to changing the culture. *'I had to accept that I would be the spokesman, the co-ordinator and the arbitrator, and really take the flak for anything that did go wrong'.*

Nurses were relieved by the new approach, once they felt able to trust it and feel safe in expressing their own fallibility.

An increase in the number of complaints caused panic initially until the team realised that this demonstrated that patients were less frightened than before. But feedback from patients remained at this stage unsatisfactory, and the unit felt it was necessary to evaluate the changes from the patients' perspective, which would also help meet the criticisms of some colleagues.

Next steps

The unit commissioned a researcher, funded by an external grant, to evaluate the nurse's role in rehabilitation and examine how the team could improve the quality of care. An action research model was chosen, since the philosophy of empowerment inherent in this approach matched that of the unit.

Data were collected over a three-year period through participant observation on the ward, and through semi-structured qualitative individual and group interviews with patients, carers, nursing staff and colleagues from other disciplines. Home interviews were carried out with 17 patients and carers. The information gathered was fed back to the ward during the project and used as a stimulus to change practice. Patients and carers were interviewed again to assess the impact of the changes by a non-nurse researcher. This meant that:

'We deliberately employed someone who was not a nurse so that they would not take things for granted. We thought we had questioned everything but quite often she asked questions we did not have the answers for. Sometimes the only answer we had was "because that is the way it has always been done". It was a frightening experience, you were really putting yourself on the line.'

The key issues that emerged were the need for information, continuity of care and help towards the empowerment of patients.

Outcomes

Empowerment of patients

Standards of care have been established, each of which starts with: *'The patient has a right to...'* These standards are audited internally and externally using observation, records and interviews with present and former patients. Interviews with patients on the ward are kept short because it is known that patients will not always voice criticism when they feel so vulnerable.

A patients' forum was set up by a primary nurse to provide both continuing feedback and an environment that would encourage patients to speak out about their care. It has proved to have a rehabilitative function as well as a consultative one – an unexpected but very positive outcome. Patients were at first reluctant to take part. Nurses needed to find ways of giving them permission and used examples of what previous patients had said to encourage them to comment, which has proved very successful.

'Patients who came to the forum meetings became far more outgoing. It has encouraged patients to move out of their own rooms more and visit each other . . .' (Clarke & Sheppard, 1992)

The forum meets between 4 pm and 6 pm, when patients are not involved in other activities and lasts for up to 50 minutes. It is patient-oriented, sometimes acting as a support group, at other times raising issues. When issues are raised that are outside the nursing staff's control, managers are brought in. For some managers, this has been the first time that they have dealt directly with patients.

'Managers are far removed from patients and have the idea that elderly people are confused, do not know what they want and probably do not need to be listened to. When the manager came to talk to people, he realised they had points of view.'

This comment arose in relation to meals, which are always an issue. The catering manager was brought in to listen to patients complaints, which had been ignored previously when raised by nurses. He said that he thought it was just the nurses who always had something to complain about. But when he heard the complaints directly from patients, things changed. The patients made him understand that little things made a lot of difference, like warming plates. But they also helped him to realise that mealtimes were a highlight of their day.

Some problems raised at the forum were easily remedied, such as a door banging in the night which had caused a lot of irritation but had been regarded as too trivial to mention. Others were far more complex and involved environmental considerations – for example, patients who had had an amputation wanted somewhere to put the prosthesis when using the toilet.

A newsletter is regularly circulated to feed back action to patients and ex-patients on longer-term issues raised in the forum. The newsletter told them, for example, how the general reluctance to use the rehabilitation garden had been overcome. Some patients feared they would not be heard from the garden, so they were given pendants to wear which linked up to a call-bell system.

The increase in the number of complaints, which the unit regards as demonstrating a successful change in culture, has led to renegotiation with the purchasers on success criteria. Former patients now link with the patient advocacy service of Brighton Healthcare and have written about the unit.

Information

Results from the action research work showed that patients and carers had not fully understood the philosophy of the ward and sometimes had unrealistic expectations. *'They expected to make a complete recovery and that a team of professionals would make them better.'*

The ward was geared towards helping patients become as independent as possible, supporting them emotionally as much as physically. The patients came from a generation that was used to seeing nurses doing things. They sometimes felt that nurses were negligent if they did not rush to help with everyday tasks. The patients needed more explanation about the ward's philosophy and why it was necessary for nurses to know when not to help as well as when they should.

To be actively involved with their care, the patients needed to be fully informed, from the beginning of their rehabilitation.

'Some things we thought we were doing well, such as giving information to patients, we found we did well on the first day of admission. We gave written information which had been discussed with previous patients ... But a lot of patients said that they had never been given the information. That came as quite a blow.'

Research showed that patients went through a huge culture shock on entering the unit, which meant they could absorb information only after they had settled in, usually after the first 48 hours. The team concluded that patients needed to be told what to expect more often and their understanding needed to be explored on a regular basis.

Patients are now given an up-to-date copy of the forum newsletter which helps them to understand the open culture of the ward and encourages them to say what they feel. However, follow-up interviews have showed that there is still a gap between the philosophy of the ward and patients' understanding of it. Staff now visit patients to tell them about the unit at the time a referral is made.

The research also showed that few patients could identify their primary nurse. Only two out of 11 patients could do so when they were asked at home, although four out of five carers could. This might have been caused partly by the no-uniform policy, which meant that patients needed more explanation about its purpose. It was also concluded that patients might recognise their own primary nurse more readily if the photographs of the team on the wall were lowered to wheelchair level and nurses' individual badges were clearer.

Continuity of care

Many of the issues identified by the research were already known to the unit – for example, the difficulties some patients found in sleeping.

Patients lying awake at night felt at their most vulnerable and were reluctant to ask for help. To provide continuity and encourage the night team in the development work, a number of action meetings were held with night staff, which led to the introduction of internal rotation.

Discharge was another issue. Both patients and carers thought the care offered in hospital was good but found the move back to the community traumatic. Carers felt that they had not been involved enough in the rehabilitation programme in hospital to be able to cope when their dependants returned home. It was realised that more needed to be done to involve carers in hospital care.

For patients, going home was difficult because of the different support they received. In hospital, as patients became more mobile, staff withdrew physical support to encourage independence, but increased psychological support. That emotional support was lower in the community, although some patients still felt in need, inevitably, several months after discharge. It was recognised that services between hospital and the community should be co-ordinated more smoothly and work is now under way to this end.

Practice

Reviews of previous research and patient response have led to continuing development work on areas such as reminiscence groups, use of music, wound dressing and other issues in which user involvement is crucial.

Reminiscence work is now part of the primary nursing role, ensuring continuity and follow-up. The right of patients to choose whether to take part or not is recognised. One of the benefits of reminiscence in rehabilitation work is that patients become the experts, reversing the usual roles. Reminiscence groups have helped some patients find the strength required to cope with the onset of disability by bringing back coping strategies adopted in the past for difficult experiences.

The therapeutic value of music was also identified from the literature. From a survey and discussion, music was found to be important to patients, particularly during the long periods of the day when they were passive.

'One after another talked knowledgeably and at great length about the music they loved. Some talked about the instruments they had played. Others described the concerts they had attended … I realised how very little I had known about my patients and their lives.'

Some said piped music was an added stress in an already stressful environment, so the unit bought personal stereos and a range of tapes, and encouraged patients to bring their own music into hospital. (Bettiss, 1993)

The onset of disability and loss of a limb were known to be traumatic for patients, but neither nurses nor doctors had the time to discuss the implications with each patient. Training, in counselling skills was identified as a priority, and the unit now has access to a clinical psychologist who can offer counselling to both patients and nurses when dealing with this issue.

It was found that staff and patients had different views about wound management. Staff knew that modern dressings often meant that wounds needed to be dressed only once a week. Patients were worried that the wound might fester and smell. In order to overcome their fears and help them understand the properties of the new dressing, patients were taught how to do their own dressings, with the view that, once discharged, they could do these dressings at home. A primary nurse became a wound specialist for this purpose.

Discussions also revealed that there were problems about the management of continence. Patients found using a catheter embarrassing and uncomfortable, but had not complained before, and even though the team thought that they gave clear explanations this was not the view of the patients. In their eyes: *'No one had explained to them why it was being done and what was being done. No one had explained that it might only be a temporary measure, and no one had asked them whether it was uncomfortable. They had not complained but had fears, about the catheter coming out.'* Staff now work with patients to find ways to make it less embarrassing and uncomfortable and have recognised that ensuring they are aware of how patients experience things is a key priority.

Lessons learned

The lessons learned from this work have had a profound effect on the team. Below is a list of the issues which now influence the way the team works:

- Don't think you know how patients and carers feel – **ask**
- Don't think you know how staff feel – **ask**
- Research takes **time**, needs **support**, requires **resources**

- Work must be **on-going, relevant, accessible**
- Significant people **must** be involved at all stages
- The **change process** takes a very long **time.**

Issues raised

While the patients' forum has proved successful, it has raised the issue of staff time. To prepare for meetings, chair them and clear up afterwards demand between three and five hours a week, and it has proved impossible for on-duty nurses to find the time.

Changing cultures and challenging established practices can be uncomfortable and can give rise to rumours if not fully explained and understood by both staff and patients.

Offering choice can raise ethical issues about consent and user involvement. These need to be openly discussed. For example, Homeward received a formal complaint from the nephew of a patient who insisted on wearing the same clothes for three days running.

The real resource constraints which exist need to be acknowledged, and this can include user involvement. The patients' forum was used to talk about how the nurses' day was organised as well as the patients' day. This helped patients to understand the resource constraints.

Contributor

Brenda Hawkey, Clinical Leader, Homeward NDU

Useful resources

Bettiss C. Caution: Music at work. Elderly Care 1993; 5(1).

Clarke M, Sheppard B. From Patient to Person. In Black G (ed). Nursing Development Units: Work in progress. London: King's Fund Centre, 1992.

Sheppard B. Homeward Bound. Health Service Journal 1994; 20(Oct):28-29.

Sheppard B. Looking Back – Moving Forward. Developing elderly care rehabilitation and the nurse's role within it. Brighton: Brighton Health Care NHS Trust, 1994.

Introducing user involvement: some practical guidelines

These guidelines are based on both the practical experiences of the five NDUs described in this booklet, and some of the literature currently available on user involvement and participation. Common principles are that individual methods will necessarily differ according to particular contexts. The following issues will be useful as a starting point for genuine involvement of users in practice.

1 Genuine involvement and partnership will take time and commitment to achieve.
Involving people is a valid aim in itself and not something that can be taken for granted in the pursuit of other goals. It is a process: how it happens is as important as the end result. Therefore it is important that people are able to decide how they want to be involved and what they want to gain from it. This is particularly pertinent to patients and carers who may feel vulnerable and grateful for the care they receive. An essential prerequisite when setting off on the path of user involvement is that there is clarity regarding: (a) your own goals; (b) the goals of the users with whom you are working; and (c) the differences between the two. This will offer a starting point on which to base your plan for development. It is important to remember that users may be somewhat reticent in offering criticism of the services offered and, as a consequence of that, their suggestions for change may be quite small at first. Success in changing these small things may be seen as the building blocks to greater involvement of users in the future.

Beresford and Croft[21] have suggested that the following points should be taken into consideration to allow involvement to take place:

- Building on the experiences that users already have will promote a patient focus to any changes.
- There is a need to be aware of the danger of unintentionally imposing one's own agenda.

- There is a need to recognise nursing skills and knowledge, without assuming that others, especially users of the service, share that knowledge.
- Sharing information; listening and providing support; enabling people to feel confident to work with staff and finally sensitivity to the fears and uncertainties of patients, carers and relatives, are crucial in developing a climate where user involvement can grow.

2 An awareness is needed regarding possible constraints to user involvement.

Change can be frightening for both staff and users. Therefore it is important that everyone involved feels they have something to contribute and to gain from the process. Keeping people informed will permit better communication between all concerned.

A lack of resources may constrain larger projects being developed, such as when extra personnel is needed to carry out a particular piece of work. However, many small changes were made within the NDUs without any extra resources which had a significant inpact on patient care.

When people feel disempowered, this will limit user involvement, and it is helpful to consider the reasons why this may be so. Bateson [22] has suggested that people feel disempowered when they do not have the information they need; when they feel confused; when they are ignored; when they are patronised; when they do not feel in control; when their experiences are devalued; and when they are stereotyped. A discussion with carers, patients, relatives and staff on these issues may go a long way in helping to promote Gibson's[23] description of empowerment as *'a process of helping people to assert control over the factors which affect their health'*.

It may be difficult for nurses to share control with users consistently. Offering choice will raise organisational issues which need to be addressed – for example, the times things are done or matters regarding the environment. Opening up discussion among staff about how care may empower or disempower users may lead to a more enquiring approach to nursing practice.

3 All staff, patients, carers and relatives should be offered the opportunity to be involved in the planning of patient participation, recognising that the climate which helps user involvement to flourish is one of partnership and collaboration.

User involvement will often mean taking risks and managing conflicts and challenges. A supportive environment, where it is safe to take risks and people are not afraid that they will be scapegoated if things go wrong, is important. User involvement may challenge the status of professionals as 'having all the answers' and may open up traditional practices to question. For most organisations this involves a considerable shift in culture. Involving staff, patients, carers and relatives is a crucial step to achieving ownership of the changes. For example, having a written philosophy of care which is widely disseminated may open up the way for criticism. However, a clear rationale will enable you to justify the changes. This is a positive step of opening up the culture of the organisation and helping to empower staff to work in new ways.

4 Units need management support to implement and to maintain user involvement initiatives.

Management support was important in all five case studies to the development of user involvement within services. In some places managers took the initiative, while in others their support had to be gained. Gaining ownership of the work within the organisation is an essential step which may be approached in a number of different ways. Some of the teams networked outside for ideas and resources as well as devising strategies for gaining ownership internally. A starting point may be establishing who is likely to be sympathetic to the work. In the case studies efforts were made to change the culture so that complaints were seen as a positive tool for change and an indication of a more open culture. This involved organisational change and as such required managerial support. For a unit to operate a successful system of user involvement, the practical commitment of staff within the unit should be matched by the political commitment of the Trust. Nevertheless, there is much which can be done at a clinical level for practitioners to initiate user involvement without waiting for more formal strategies.

5 Involving users should take place in both informal and formal ways within organisations.

Formal messages send clear indications to users that their involvement is sought. However, this can sometimes be tokenistic. For example, it is quite demoralising for patients to be asked to fill in a questionnaire in an outpatients' department and go back for another appointment to find that changes to the service offered have not taken place. Informal work usually consists of participation in a more immediate way and is likely to have a more direct effect on the care which people receive, such as changing the pillow covers at Weston Park (see p.38), but may not be legitimised within the organisation.

It may also help to undertake an audit of the work already being carried out throughout the organisation. Initiatives may be listed under user involvement, patient participation or advocacy. Establishing what has been learned from this work and how it could be taken forward may prove to be valuable in setting priorities for user involvement. It may help to link up with voluntary or self-help groups who can feed into development plans and may be able to lobby particular individuals within your organisation in order to gain support for your ideas.

Users should be involved at different levels of the organisation on the range of concerns and decisions that are made on both service and treatment issues. Analysing where decisions are made within your organisation may highlight where user involvement would be critical to help change services. Identifying the resources that users may need, such as training, administrative support or expenses, and making sure that these resources are provided will go a long way in legitimising the user's position.

6 Support, training and resourcing are usually required for user involvement to take place at all levels of the organisation. According to the degree of involvement, both users and staff will need training.

Users

Sometimes it will be enough for users to bring their experiences to whatever forum is being planned. At other times users and carers may need to be offered training or preparation to enable them to be part of a formal structure. If, for instance, there is an expectation that users need to contribute to strategic committee meetings then it is critical to assess their needs regarding training in committee skills. Practical support systems will need to be set up for users to be involved which may include payment of expenses, access to a telephone and photocopying, help with childcare or other caring responsibilities while attending meetings. This will allow users to contribute actively and go some way in valuing their contributions. Who will carry out and resource this training needs to be established as does the setting-up of a support system for users. The local community health council may be able to offer help with this.

Staff

Training will allow staff to discuss honestly what needs to change, what prevents change and share ideas on how to move forward. Service users, where possible, should be used in this training, making sure they are paid at the same rate as other trainers. Bringing in someone external to the unit can offer a fresh perspective on how to move forward with development plans. It is important to be aware of the fears among staff regarding new working practices. The establishment of good supervision and support will be necessary.

7 Communicating good, relevant information is a prerequisite to user involvement.

Most information available has tended to concentrate on service issues but there is a need to expand this into treatment areas. Some people want practical information while others may want to be involved in decision making. Ascertaining what level of information people want demands skilful judgement. In some contexts negotiation of information giving will be central to the overall care of patients. Disagreements between professionals sometimes means that information for users is bland and not particularly relevant. Offering choice, particularly in treatment, will mean making some of the areas of uncertainty within health care more explicit.

Research consistently shows that users want more information about all areas of health care which affect them, including areas of uncertainty, and that professionals underestimate the amount of information that users want.[24, 25]

Hogg[26] identified a continuum of information as follows:

INFORMATION ABOUT...	INFORMATION TO HELP PEOPLE TO:	USER INVOLVEMENT
Services available • What services are available • How to use services	Use services better	PASSIVE ↑
Education • Health education on: – life style – specific conditions and diseases – specific operations/treatments	Improve health by following advice of professionals	│
Self help groups • Self help groups • Self care after diagnosis or treatment	Manage the condition better	│
Clinical • What standards to expect • Clinical performance/complication rates etc. • Effects and side effects of drugs/treatments • Choices of treatment	Make choices and decisions	↓ ACTIVE

Source: C Hogg. *Beyond the Patient's Charter.* London: Health Rights Ltd, 1994. Reproduced by permission.

In order to achieve what Hogg suggests, finding out what information is already available, followed by consultation with carers and users regarding how helpful and relevant it is, needs to be seen as a priority. Together with this there is a need to determine whether the information received was given at the appropriate time.

Information needs of particular client groups should be taken into consideration – for example, providing information on tape as well as leaflets will permit those who have sensory impairments to access the information. It is also necessary to have the information available in different community languages.

Effective information-giving is a difficult area to get right, therefore a list of suggested reading appears at the back of the book which may help people to consider a way forward on this issue.

8 It is necessary to identify and discuss the ethical dilemmas which user involvement may present in nursing practice.

Nursing theorists have seen patient participation as an ethical ideal. Ashworth's[27] view is that nurses should attempt to promote patient participation as a consequence of their respect for patients' autonomy as people. However, what happens when patients feel they do not want to be involved? In some situations offering choice can be perceived as negligence, as seen in Homeward NDU (see p.50), particularly by relatives and carers, if there has been insufficient explanation. Another challenge is that of questioning the traditional expectations of the public who may see offering choice and user involvement as a move away from a caring ethos.

There is no easy answers to any of these issues. What is important is that they are recognised and discussed with both patients, carers and staff so that solutions can be found. Answers should be tailored to individual patients, and this will involve skilful negotiation between nurses and patients.

It must be remembered that users, like professionals, are not a homogenous group and have conflicting views and interests. This needs to be acknowledged from the outset and a forum must be provided which permits flexibility in addressing particular areas of concern.

9 **There is no one methodology which is appropriate for all settings. Often a combination of different approaches is most successful. Once the goals of all concerned have been identified, then it is possible to match these to appropriate methods.**
Not all methods of involvement suit all groups. It is therefore important to consider a range of options.

Questionnaires are commonly used to elicit information from users of services. Although there are advantages, they are not always the most appropriate method for approaching users. They can exclude particular groups from participating, such as those whose first language is not English or people with sensory impairments or learning difficulties. If questionnaires are devised by professionals, excluding users, there is a risk that they only represent a preset agenda, without including the most important information that users may have to offer.

Gathering information on relevant work already carried out will avoid duplication. Some literature can be obtained from voluntary organisations, community health councils and self-help groups. For example, in mental health, MIND have a useful set of guidelines on user involvement.[28]

When considering methods, attention should be given to those groups of users whose views and experiences have historically been under-represented within health services. For example, feedback from black and minority ethnic communities should inform the development of a health and race strategy.[29] Women may be the majority of users in the health service but their views and concerns as women may not be represented adequately. Equally, it is important to ensure that methods are used which do not prevent disabled people from participating in all aspects of user involvement. Lesbian women and gay men who use the services can also face negative attitudes which may prevent them from expressing their specific concerns.

Interviews, discussion groups or advisory groups comprising users or representatives of self-help organisations are all helpful in exploring what the user's agenda is. The information gained can then be fed into a management process which allows those providing care to discover the users' views of the service which is currently offered.

Investigation will be required in each unit before decisions on how to best involve users can be taken. Many methods which have been used in different settings can be replicated. For example, advocacy can be used in a range of settings, not just mental health.

10 Work needs to be ongoing, with the relevant results fed back to users and staff. Regular monitoring and evaluation systems should be integral to the process with input from all concerned, including users.

The feeding back of results from studies undertaken is essential in gaining users' commitment to carry out further work. An openness in feeding back information to users may go some way to avoiding confusion about decisions which have been made.

Monitoring user involvement initiatives will involve the use of appropriate monitoring tools. These may range from organisational monitoring, such as keeping detailed minutes of meetings or making financial information available to users, to more sophisticated monitoring or audit on qualitative issues, such as the actual experiences users have had of the service.

Alternatively, users could carry out the evaluation of involvement initiatives by drawing up questionnaires, carrying out interviews and analysing the data collected.

Other approaches which can be taken to monitor effectiveness include patient or carer forums, pre-defined audit tools or focus groups.

References

1. Department of Health. The Patient's Charter. London: HMSO, 1991.

2. NHSME. Local Voices. London: NHS Management Executive, 1992.

3. Department of Health. Caring for People. London: HMSO, 1989.

4. Cartwright A. The Dignity of Labour? London: Tavistock, 1979.

5. Green J M, Coupland V A, Kitzinger J V. Great Expectations: A prospective study of women's expectations and experiences of childbirth. Cambridge: Child Care and Development Group, 1988.

6. Green J M, Coupland V A, Kitzinger J V. Expectations, experiences and psychological outcomes of childbirth. Birth 1990; 17:15-24.

7. Jacoby A. Women's preferences for and satisfaction with current procedures in childbirth. Findings from a national study. Midwifery 1987; 3:117-24

8. Department of Health. Changing Childbirth. London: HMSO, 1993.

9. McIver S. Obtaining the Views of Users of Health Services. London: King' Fund Centre, 1991.

10. Hall J A, Dornan M C. What patients like about their medical care and how often they are asked: A meta analysis of satisfaction literature. Social Science and Medicine 1988; 27:935-9.

11. Dixon P, Carr Hill R A. Consumer satisfaction surveys: A review. The NHS and its customers. York: Centre for Health Economics, 1989.

12. Carr Hill R A. The measurement of patient satisfaction. Journal of Public Health Medicine 1992; 14:3.

13. Bruster S, Jarman B, Bosanquet N *et al.* National survey of hospital patients. British Medical Journal 1994; 309:1542-6.

14. Sykes W, Collins M, Hunter D *et al.* Listening to Local Voices: A guide to research methods. Leeds: Nuffield Institute, 1992.

15. Williams G, Popay J. Researching the People's Health: Dilemmas and opportunities for social scientists. Salford: Public Health Research and Resource Centre, 1992.

16. Cochrane A L. Effectiveness and Efficiency. Random reflections on health services. Leeds: Nuffield Provincial Hospital Trust, 1971.

17. Coulter A. Assembling the evidence – Outcomes research. In Dunning M, Needham G (eds). But Will It Work Doctor? Winchester: Consumer Health Information Consortium, 1994.

18. Kelleher D. Self-help groups and their relationship to medicine. In: Gabe J, Kelleher D, Williams G (eds). Challenging Medicine. London: Routlege, 1994.

19. Gurney B H. Public Participation in Health Care, A Critical Review of the Issues and Methods. Cambridge: East Anglian Regional Health Authority, 1994.

20. Glenister H. Patient participation in psychiatric services: A literature review and proposal for a research strategy. Journal of Advanced Nursing 1994; 19:802-11.

21. Beresford P, Croft S. Citizen Involvement: A practical guide for change. Basingstoke: Macmillan, 1993.

22. Bateson B. Empowerment. In: The public as partners, a tool box for involving people in commissioning health care. Cambridge: Cambridge Health Authority, 1992.

23. Gibson C H. A concept analysis of empowerment. Journal of Advanced Nursing 1991; 16(3):354-61

24. McIver S. Obtaining the Views of Users of Health Services about Quality of Information. London: King's Fund Centre, 1993.

25. Audit Commission. What seems to be the matter? Communication between hospitals and patients. London: HMSO, 1993.

26. Hogg C. Beyond the Patient's Charter. Working with users: a practical guide for people working in the health service. London: Health Rights, 1994.

27. Ashworth P D, Longmate M A, Morrison P. Patient participation: Its meaning and significance in the context of caring. Journal of Advanced Nursing 1992; 17:1430-9.

28. MIND. The MIND Guide to Advocacy in Mental Health: Empowerment in action. London: MIND, 1992.

29. Gunaratnam Y. Checklist Health and Race: A starting point for managers on improving services for black populations. London: King's Fund Centre, 1993.

Further reading

User involvement

Beresford P, Croft S. Citizen Involvement: A practical guide for change. Basingstoke: Macmillan, 1993.

Britchie J, Wann M. Training for lay participation in health, token voices or champions of the people? London: Patients' Association, 1992.

Fielder B, Twitchin D. Achieving User Participation. Planning services for people with severe physical and sensory disabilities. Living Options in Practice Project Paper No. 3. London: King's Fund Centre, 1992.

Health Gain Standing Conference. The public as partners, a tool-box for involving people in commissioning health care. Cambridge: Cambridge Health Authority, 1992.

Hogg C. Beyond the Patient's Charter. London: Health Rights, 1993.

Jamdagni L. The tale of the chapatti maker. King's Fund News 1994: 17(Winter):3-4.

McIver S. An Introduction to Obtaining the Views of Users of Health Services. London: King's Fund Centre, 1991.

McIver S. Obtaining the Views of Users of Mental Health Services. London: King's Fund Centre, 1991.

McIver S. Obtaining the Views of Inpatients and Users of Casualty Departments. London: King's Fund Centre, 1992.

McIver S. Obtaining the Views of Users of Primary and Community Health Care Services. London: King's Fund Centre, 1993.

McIver S. Obtaining the Views of Black Users of Health Services. London: King's Fund Centre, 1994.

Rigge M. Involving patients and consumers. The Health Service Journal: Health Management Guide, 18 October 1993.

Sheppard B. Looking back – Moving forward. Developing elderly care rehabilitation and the nurse's role within it. Brighton: Brighton Health Care NHS Trust, 1994.

Unwin L (ed). Power to the People: The key to responsive services in health and social care. London: King's Fund Centre, 1990.

Whittaker A, Gardner S, Kershaw J. Service Evaluation by People with Learning Difficulties. London: King's Fund Centre, 1991.

Information

Audit Commission. What seems to be the matter. Communication between hospitals and patients. London: HMSO, 1993.

Gann B, Needham G. Promoting Choice. Consumer Health Information in the 1990's. Winchester: Help for Health Trust, 1991.

McIver S. Obtaining the Views of Users of Health Services about Quality of Information. London: King's Fund Centre, 1993.

Relevant legislation and guidance

NHSME. Local Voices. London, NHS Management Executive, 1992.

Department of Health. Caring for People. London: HMSO, 1989.

Department of Health. The Patient's Charter. London: HMSO, 1991.

Department of Health. Working for Patients. London: HMSO, 1991.

World Health Organization. Health for All 2000. Copenhagen: WHO, 1978.

Research issues

Barnes M, Wistow G (eds). Researching User Involvement. Seminar series. The Nuffield Institute for Health Services Studies. University of Leeds, 1992.

Popay J, Williams G. Researching the People's Health. London: Routledge, 1994.

Sykes W, Collins M, Hunter D *et al.* Listening to Local Voices. A guide to research methods. Nuffield Institute for Health Services Studies: Public Health Research and Resource Centre, 1992.

Organisational change

Handy C. Understanding Organisations. 3rd e. New York: Facts on File, 1985.

Kanter R M. The Change Masters: Corporate entrepreneurs at work. London: Allen & Unwin, 1984.

Menzies I E P. The functioning of social systems as a defence against anxiety. Human Relation 1960; 13:95-121.

Health and race

Ahmad W I U (ed). Race and health in contemporary Britain. Buckingham: Open University Press, 1993.

Health Education Authority. Health-Related Resources for Black and Minority Ethnic Groups. London: HEA, 1994.

Health Education Authority. Black and Minority Ethnic Groups in England: Health and lifestyles. London: HEA, 1994.

Mares P, Henley A, Baxter C. Health Care in Multiracial Britain. London: HEA, 1985.

Outcomes

Dunning M, Needham G. But Will It Work Doctor? Winchester: Consumer Health Information Consortium, 1994.

Involving users in quality and audit

National Consumer Council. Quality Standards in the NHS, the consumer focus. London: NCC, 1992.

Pfeffer N, Coote A. Is Quality Good For You? A critical review of quality assurance in welfare services. London: Institute for Public Policy Research, 1991.